MORNING ROUTINE

3 Simple Steps to Energize Yourself and Stay Motivated During the Day

By CARRIE DRESDEN

Table of Contents

Introduction

Chances are, if you are looking to wake up early, you have read countless articles on the best way to achieve this. It seems like such an easy thing to achieve, but as we all know, it can be a huge struggle day in and day out. If you are aiming to get up early, and you are looking for the tips, tricks and advice to really make the change and start getting up early on a regular basis, then this is definitely the book for you.

This is the ultimate morning routine blueprint, which will guide you to morning routine mastery. It will help you for sure with the process of creating morning routine checklist and will guide you to higher productivity and positive thinking.

In this book, we cover a range of ideas, methods and more, to ensure that you get up early once and for all. Unlike most posts, which mainly focus on the action plan, we will be focusing on both practical implementations, as well as the deeper motivation that definite whether you truly get out of bed at the time you intended too. This includes focusing on willpower, the greater reason why you want to get out of bed earlier, and visualization.

If you follow all of the tips in this book and stick with them, we can guarantee that you will be able to get up early on a daily basis WITHIN A WEEK. Just stick with the habit, follow our easy instructions, and we know that you will find the success that you have been working towards for such a long time.

Chapter 1: Determine Your Why

The title of this book has got to do with creating a fantastic morning routine that ensures you get where you want to go, and stay energized and productive throughout the day. Out of all the habits and pieces of information on doing this, the most important habit and aspect of a successful morning routine is waking up early. This does not mean waking up at 5 am every day if you're used to waking up at 10am, but it does mean waking up earlier than you usually do, and making the most of that time. Maybe you work late as a bartender, and waking up at 5am is just not going to happen for you. This doesn't mean that waking early doesn't apply to you. There are ways to ensure you wake up earlier than you usually do and use this time productively and joyfully. This is how so many people find that success that they do.

So, while this book talks about morning routine, we would like to stress now that the most important part is waking up early, and formulating your routine around that. In this book, we will talk about overcoming the challenges of waking up, and how you can use this to your advantage and ensure that you get the most out of each and every day that you have on this earth. If you want to write that book and get it done, if you want to start your own business, start running, have more time for yourself, enjoy life more, of anything else, then this book is for you! Rather than talking about what you should be doing, or what you should spend every minute on, we will give you concrete strategies that you can apply no matter what your goal is, or how you want to continue forward. Be it a plan to finally get rich, or a plan to spend more time with your children, if you follow the steps in this chapter, and the rest of the book, you will most certainly find success in the very best way, in a joyful way that is free of the stress you hate.

Waking up early has so many positive benefits, such as increased energy, decreased stress, increased productivity and so much more. By doing this, you will find strength and energy that you did not even know existed, and easily transform your life into one that you enjoy, and are excited about each and every day. This is a fantastic thought, and if you are anything like me, this will spur you on like nothing else.

Everyone would like more enjoyment, more time, more energy and to get things done faster- this is the benefit that waking earlier can do for you, and is why we touch on it so heavily in this chapter and the chapters ahead. Even though it is usually considered a difficult skill to learn, we believe that anyone can do it will a little practice, time, and encouragement.

One of the biggest reasons that people fail in their plan to start waking up early is the fact that they do not know their deeper motivation. Often, waking up early is just something that we think we should do, because all of the most successful people do it, or it is seen as a great habit to have. It is important to realize that we should not focus on what society says we should do, since this is very rarely good motivation. Instead, we end up feeling pressured, guilty and like we are failing at some fundamental level. This is a horrible way to feel and it does nothing for you or your motivation.

In fact, guilt rarely works to do anything but make us feel horrible, and this is not effective in the slightest.

So how should we go about it instead? It is very important to determine exactly what you are working towards and aiming towards by waking up early. This can be anything from hoping to have a more peaceful morning, hoping to be more organized, or working on a special project. It is different for everyone, and everyone has a completely different opinion, goal, and purpose in life. This is why it is important to find out exactly why you want to get up early. One of the most challenging parts of doing this is the fact that you probably want to conform to societal standards quite quickly. The idea that pops to your mind first is probably one that you have heard a hundred times before, and you may not really believe in. You need to ensure that you really know why you want to wake up early, and if you don't have a reason, then you need to find one.

Maybe you want to wake up so that you can read your book and drink some tea. This is not exactly a productive idea, but it might light your fire and be the reason to get out of bed. You can then use this momentum to work on more productive things later. This can be a great way to enjoy the time you have, and motivate you to get out of bed.

So how do you go about finding out the reason that you want to get out of bed? One great way to do this is to simply write it out, write out a long, long stream of ideas, things you enjoy, what is important to you, and so much more. Eventually, you will come across something that makes you smile. This is the reason you should wake up earlier and is a fantastic way to brighten up your morning.

Once you have determined why you want to get up earlier, you need to ensure that you don't forget it. If possible, make it part of your alarm, a song that reminds you or your goal, or something along those lines. You need to make sure that you have it up somewhere that you can see it, on the fridge, the notice board, or somewhere else. This is very important and can help you increase your motivation and succeed in ways that you could never have imagined before.

Make sure you put it up in multiple places, write it in your diary, make it your screensaver and whatever else you can do to keep this information in the very front of your mind so that you see it constantly and are always reminded of what you are working towards. This is an awesome way of making sure that you are always thinking about your goal, planning for it and working on it. Once you have this down, I can guarantee that you will find much more success before, just with this simple step. There is, however, the next step to this.

Once you have determined the reason why you want to get up so early, you can often use this to your advantage even further. The night before, make sure that you set up your workstation, your reading station, or whatever else you plan to do. Make it an utter priority to set up this area. This ties in heavily with making sure you remember yours why. By using the night before to prepare for it, you will have no excuse in the morning. Perhaps you can set out your running shoes, or set your coffee machine to brew that perfect cup at the time you want to get up. Whatever goal you are working towards, and whatever you have decided your ideal morning goal is, you need to make it accessible as possible the night before, so that you will have no trouble at all sorting through the information in your head when you wake up. Your excuses will be minimized and you will have a far greater chance of success.

It is quite a little thing and something that many people overlook in favor of conforming and making sure that their goals look good, but it is such an important step to wake up for what you truly love. This is what will bring the smile to your face, and set your day off right. This is better than forcing yourself into something you hate right away. Take time to do what you enjoy, or what motivates you and has you burning with energy and passion. This is how you will succeed in the very best ways, and this is a fantastic first step for anyone who is working hard towards achieving their goal of finally, finally getting up early come hell or high water.

So if you are unclear on your why, or you don't really have one yet, then please, please do not skip this step. It is easily the most important step on the list, and can skyrocket you forward into the success that you need, desire and deserve.

By taking a few minutes to write it out and plan, you will be setting the rest of your day, week, month and life up for more success than you could ever imagine!

Chapter 2: Plan

We touched on this one briefly in the last chapter, but it cannot be stressed enough! Planning is one of the most important ingredients when it comes to waking up early. This extends to pretty much every part of your life, and every part of the process of waking up.

You need to plan to go to bed at a reasonable time in order to ensure you have the energy to wake up early and make it through the day. There is no point in going to bed late, waking up early and then finding yourself too exhausted to get anything done at all. This is a stressful and horrible way to live, and the way to avoiding this starts by planning to go to bed early.

Once you have made the decision to go to bed early, you need to plan a number of other aspects of your life. For example, if you are planning to go to bed early, you may have to adjust the way you are working at the moment. If you are used to having dinner at a late hour, you will need to adjust it to a more reasonable time in order for your food to digest properly. If you are used to drinking coffee well into the afternoon, then you need to change this in order to ensure that you have the time to properly process the caffeine and ensure you have a restful sleep, instead of lying awake all night.

Not only do you have to change your own lifestyle, but you need to ensure you communicate this to your family. Maybe you are used to spending time with your partner watching TV at the end of the day. You may need to see if you can sneak away together on your lunch breaks, or if you could start the ritual a little earlier, in order to make sure you have the time you need to rest properly.

This is a big thing, and you need to plan ahead in order to make it happen. Another thing to plan is cutting down on your screen time right before bed, and planning some sort of calming ritual. This might be a warm shower, time with a book, meditation, a cup of hot chocolate, or anything else that you use to calm down and destress your mind! Unfortunately, working with screens does not soothe your mind, and is a poor way to go to sleep.

Because of this, you will have to plan a few things in your life that need to change in order to ensure that you can stick to your planned habit of waking up earlier. It is far too easy to act as if these things are inevitable and unavoidable, and let them stop you time and time again. However, they are most certainly avoidable, and you can make changes and implement different tactics in your life in order to ensure that you get this done no matter what.

That is not the only thing you need to plan in advance, though! It is important to make sure that you have a good and solid grasp of your morning routine. Make sure you have an alarm set in advance, for every single day, so that you do not forget, or accidently turn it off the night before. If you have it set every morning, you know that you can rely on it to wake you up every morning. Make sure your alarm clock is plugged in, or your phone is charged and face down so that it does not disturb your sleep or your rest. This is a good way to really get in the mindset of waking early every day. It is important that your mind knows this is a routine and not just a one-off thing. This is how you cement it within your psyche.

One you have organized your alarm, you need to have a good look at your morning routine. Have you planned it out in the best way possible? If you are aiming to get more work done, do you have an area where you can do it without disturbing your loved ones? If you plan on getting some reading done is your book set out the night before? If you want to go for a run, do you have your outfit and jogging shoes set out for you to jump into in the morning?

Make sure that you do everything in your power to make it as easy as possible for yourself, so that you do not hit constant roadblocks along the way. Planning is a fantastic way to overcome any resistance as it eliminates many of the excuses that you may have been using. Plan how you are going to use your momentum throughout the rest of the day. If you are planning on getting work done, then hitting the gym, plan what time you'll start getting ready, set an alarm on your phone, and have the next phase of the plan all ready and set for you to just get going. These are all great ways to overcome the resistance that many of us naturally feel when we are stepping out of our comfort zone. If you truly want to get this done, this is a good place to start.

So how do you start planning? Maybe you really feel like you have no idea where to start or what is holding you back. How to you start accessing how you need to change your situation? Well, much like in the previous chapter, one great way to do so is by brainstorming. Grab a journal and start writing it down bit by bit until you have a plan all set out and ready to go. You might have to write a few different drafts, but eventually, you will find the sweet spot. Once you have figured out exactly what you need to do, tackle and change, it is a fantastic idea to write yourself a checklist of some kind, so that you can easily work through your list of getting things done. By doing this, you can ensure that you really do find out every little roadblock that will get in your way.

Now, you can't plan for everything, and sometimes life happens. If you have to attend an evening event, or it is date night with your partner, you might have to let things slide now and then. It can be easy to get hung up on this as a failure, but it's not. Every now and then, life will find a way to knock you down, be it by emergency, illness or a special night out.

However, the important thing is to plan to get back on the horse once it is over. It's okay to go out to a few parties now and then, but once they are done, you need to start waking up early again. Enjoy life, and don't let this make you miserable, but remember to plan, plan, plan, and get back on the horse when life knocks you off it.

Sometimes, planning can seem like such a big mission. We think that we can just wing it and everything will work out just fine, but that is rarely the case. Usually a lack of planning results in a lack of discipline and an aimless day where you are at the whims of life. When you plan your day, you are in charge of how much you get done, and how you feel. You can choose to be happy, choose to make time for the things that you enjoy and balance your work and your life so that you have the content and satisfaction that you deserve. Truly, we cannot stress this enough. Planning your day makes sure that you have enough time for what is truly important, be that family, friends, your artwork, time to relax or more. It is very important to plan. Planning for things that might go wrong is also very important. It is easy for things to happen that might cause a spanner in the works, such as a change in location, an emergency, or something coming up at work. Once you have done your best to give yourself extra free time, you will be able to fit more into your day. It is vital to ensure you find a good balance of work and play every day.

It is this balance that brings together everything you need to know and do, in your life. It helps you grow more focused and resilient. If you start your day off on a calm, organized note, then you are so much more likely to be able to handle any negative changes that might occur within your day to day. If you get sick, you will not be as far behind, if you have to go out that evening for a meeting, or you get in a fight with your boss, you will be able to handle everything so much better if you are not only well rested, but balanced, and have planned everything you need to do. This is such a powerful way to engage in life, and planning is most certainly the very first step to doing this, no matter what you have on. This is a great way to ensure that everything goes as smoothly as you need it to. So while planning might seem hard at first, it is so, so worth it, and the benefits that it has on you, and on your family, are endless and plentiful in every single way possible.

By following these planning tips, your mornings, and your life will just go so much smoother every time! And that is a great thing.

Chapter 3: Enlist Support

If you are truly struggling to wake up early, then you might want to look at your support system. Maybe your partner doesn't get why you want to do this so badly, and is resentful of the change, and the time it takes from the relationship. Maybe your friends love to go partying every night and tease you constantly for going to bed so early.

These are very, very detrimental to your success and can be damaging to your new goal. Even if your friends and family are indifferent, this can be a painful thing to deal with as you are not getting the support that you need. One good way to deal with this is to find an alternative support system. Perhaps you can go online and find a group of people all reaching for their goals. They do not have to share the same goal, but this can be a fantastic way to really get the support and positive energy that you need. Not only that, but you can often find great accountability, the feeling that other people are counting on you to really fulfill your goals, much like you are counting on them.

This is a powerful way to motivate yourself and can really be an important step in finding that motivation. If you're not into group motivation, then seek out a friend or college who is trying to achieve something too. You can agree to motivate each other and be accountability partners. Like before, it doesn't matter if it is a different goal to your own, so long as you are both committed to your own goals and supportive of each other. It can be helpful to discuss your struggles and your successes with someone who is understanding and sympathetic.

Often, this support system is the thing we truly need for pushing us to the next level and allowing ourselves to succeed in ways that you never dreamed of before. Support is a powerful thing that can motivate you to do your best even in difficult situations. This is a good way to make sure you stay on track, even if your close friends and family are not very supportive of you.

But what if your friends and family are supportive of you? Then this is a great way to tap into their support and make sure you tell them what you are trying to achieve. If you know without a doubt that your loved ones will support you no matter what, then this is a great time to open up to them and really let them know your plans, your goals and more. This is a good accountability factor, as they will make sure you stick to the plan, by asking how you're doing. It's natural to not want to disappoint them, so you will most likely try much harder to get it right.

Of course, the benefits of letting them know do not stop there. You will find that if you let your friends and family know, they will help you in many other ways, such as scheduling earlier get-togethers, or making date night a little earlier than usual. This can be a wonderful feeling, so make sure to return the favor when your friends and family are working on their own goals.

If your partner is trying to achieve the same goal as you, then it can be a very powerful thing to work on it together. Maybe doing something fun together when you wake early, or reward each other for getting through another week. This reinforcement and support can ensure that you get there in no time. It is often so much easier to do things with someone else than alone, especially when you are working on a new habit, a new way of life, or a big change.

And after all, waking up early is a pretty big change, and should not be taken lightly by any stretch of the imagination. Now, while we are technically talking about morning routines, this is such a vital part of it that we just need to include it in this piece. After all, without support, it can feel impossible to get things done in the ways that you have always hoped to do. So next time you are struggling with a new habit, such as waking up early, this is a fantastic way to get things done and organized really well and really fast. If you are ever wondering if other successful people do this then do not fear! This is such an important part of waking up early that everyone who succeeds has some sort of support and help in getting there. After all, waking up early is deceptively simple, and many people do not realize just how challenging it can be until they experience it themselves!

Conclusion

From the chapter above, it is clear how important it is to start your morning off right by waking up early. Waking up early is the key to much of the success that we have through the rest of the day, and can set us up to have a wonderful morning.

Of course, one of the key aspects of this book is the fact that you need to get up for a good reason. You must have a powerful and important reason to get up early, one that fills you with enjoyment, happiness, and motivation. This powerful passion needs to be what fuels you onwards, as it is the most impactful and important that you could ever have. Getting up for no good reason will fill you with exhaustion and dread, and the habit is likely to die early. But if you wake up with a purpose and passion in your mind, you are sure to be filled with the sort of energy and enjoyment that will carry you through your entire day without any issues.

Below, we summarize some of the best and most important points from the book.

Once you have determined why you want to get up earlier, you need to ensure that you don't forget it. If possible, make it part of your alarm, a song that reminds you or your goal, or something along those lines. You need to make sure that you have it up somewhere that you can see it, on the fridge, the notice board, or somewhere else. This is very important and can help you increase your motivation and succeed in ways that you could never have imagined before.

Once you have made the decision to go to bed early, you need to plan a number of other aspects of your life. For example, if you are planning to go to bed early, you may have to adjust the way you are working at the moment. If you are used to having dinner at a late hour, you will need to adjust it to a more reasonable time in order for your food to digest properly. If you are used to drinking coffee well into the afternoon, then you need to change this in order to ensure that you have the time to properly process the caffeine and ensure you have a restful sleep, instead of lying awake all night.

Support is a vital part of making sure you succeed in your goal, and group motivation is a brilliant way to do it. Finding an online support or accountability group is a great way to get started. This is a powerful way to motivate yourself and can really be an important step in finding that motivation. If you're not into group motivation, then seek out a friend or college who is trying to achieve something too. You can agree to motivate each other and be accountability partners. Like before, it doesn't matter if it is a different goal to your own, so long as you are both committed to your own goals and supportive of each other. It can be helpful to discuss your struggles and your successes with someone who is understanding and sympathetic.

Through waking up early, you can find the motivation and the energy to carry you through the rest of your day. Waking up early has been linked to increased productivity and increased success rates, as well as a higher likelihood that you will be happy. Happiness is a powerful motivator and should be kept in mind. If you wake up early, you will have access to more time for yourself, more time for your projects, more time to do what you love and make your dreams come true. Things that have always felt impossible are now possible, and it is a beautiful and amazing process to be a part of, no matter what your age, gender of occupation. Through this process, you will create the life that you desire, and truly deserve, and there is nothing stopping you. You have the power, the strength, the intelligence and so much more. You can make your dreams come true, without a doubt!

If you are truly motivated to wake up early and begin your morning routine on the best foot, then this is a great way to start and truly make it work. With the strength that you find through your support network and the powerful energy that comes with knowing your why, you will be able to succeed no matter what. By planning in advance and ensuring that you have eliminated any negativity and road blocks, there is nothing to stop you from truly achieving your goal, waking up early and starting the day on an energetic and powerful note.